Ketogenic Fat Bombs

©Greg Mason

Forward

"One of the secrets of a happy life is continuous small treats" - Iris Murdoch

When we think of treats on a diet I am sure we are all thinking sweets however this is usually a staple that is highly avoided when on a diet. Each of us has some sort of treat we enjoy however most diets have had you give up some of your favorite treats. Whether it be cookies, cakes or ice creams, I am sure being on the ketogenic diet you wouldn't expect to have a whole lot of options for sweet treats.

Desserts are one of those things that just make you wonder if your diet is really worth missing out all the little pleasures that life has to offer. We often see sweet treats as obstacles that we tend to steer clear of once we are on a diet. However if you are like me I am sure that the temptation to have a sweet treat is more than vivid in your thoughts no matter how hard you try to stay away from those 'unhealthy' foods. I don't think anyone can resist a sweet treat but sometimes we end up feeling bad after we have indulge. Well I think we can turn that frown upside down because do I have some good news for you.

You are about to be the happiest you could ever be. Did I mention ketogenic diet is amazing! Desserts are here to stay with you on the ketogenic diet and you won't have any need to feel guilty when you have them. You can still have cakes and ice cream too and best of all you can make them all yourself. That's right you can have sweet treats on the keto journey.

In this book, we share with you a variety of mouthwatering, ketogenic sweet treats that come together quickly and easily! These recipes are all ketogenic approved and are sure to satisfy your sweet tooth.

Whether you're new to the ketogenic diet and wondering what type of foods to eat, or a ketogenic diet veteran who needs some inspiration, this book is here to help!

As you embark on this health journey, I hope it leads you to a life of pure health bliss and vitality as it has for so many ketogenic devotees.

I hope you enjoy this book and the decadent recipes herein, as it was definitely one of my favorite projects to work on. Bon appetite!

Table of Contents

3

Overview of the Ketogenic Diet

The ketogenic diet can be a most rewarding experience for anyone that chooses to stick with it. In case you aren't familiar with the diet, here's a brief overview:

The ketogenic diet is a low carb, high fat diet that allows your body to be put into a state of ketosis where your body targets fat as its source of energy. Though you consume more fats than the norm these are used up quite quickly by the body. We normally get our energy from carbohydrates however on the ketogenic diet there is minimal intake of carbohydrates and thus the body targets the greatest source that it has which is fats.

Just bear in mind that they body will not be storing the added intake of fat that you will now be eating thus resulting in the weight loss and a healthier body. Now how exactly will eating fats make you healthier? Your body will be in a constant state of ketosis and this is where you are tricking your body into thinking it is hungry. You won't ever actually feel hungry in this diet though. Whenever your body is hungry it targets your energy source to keep your body functioning. On a 'normal' diet this source would be carbohydrates but in a state of ketosis this source is now fats.

Now if you are diabetic and have a real concern about consuming carbohydrates then this is the perfect diet for you as carbohydrates are kept to a minimum. Many diabetic persons have reported that their conditions have been improved or been rid of by being on the ketogenic diet. The ketogenic diet is for type 2 diabetics only or for some persons suffering with epilepsy. As with any diet it is important to discuss issues or concerns you may have with a physician before starting.

But since this is a deserts recipe book I am sure there is cause for concern about sweets. However be reassured that all ingredients in these recipes are tailored for you if you are diabetic. These may be substituted with whatever brand you favor. There's no need to feel very restricted on the ketogenic diet as you can already tell by the fact that desserts are included. You will soon no longer refer to the ketogenic diet as a diet but as a lifestyle. You can share your recipes with persons who are not on the keto journey too and I'm sure you'll have no complaints.

Recipes

Coconut Cashew Bars

Serves 8

Ingredients

Almond flour (1 cup)

Maple syrup (1/4 cup, sugar free)

Salt (to taste)

Coconut (1/4 cup, shredded)

Butter (1/4 cup, melted)

Cinnamon (1 teaspoon)

Cashews (1/2 cup)

Directions

1. Put flour and butter in a bowl and mix together thoroughly.
2. Add coconut, salt, cinnamon and syrup to flour mixture and combine.
3. Add cashews to mixture and thoroughly mix.
4. Use parchment paper to line a baking sheet and add cashew mixture to the sheet and spread evenly.
5. Refrigerate for 2 hours or more.
6. Slice and serve.

Nutritional Information

Calories 189

Net Carbs 4g

Fats 17.6g

Protein 4g

Fiber 2.1g

Keto Peanut Butter Chocolate Tarts

Serves 8

Ingredients

For Crust:

Flaxmeal (1/4 cup)

Erythritol (1 tablespoon)

Almond flour (2 tablespoons)

Egg white (1)

For top Layer:

Cocoa powder (4 tablespoons)

Vanilla (1/2 teaspoon)

Heavy cream (2 tablespoons)

Avocado (1)

Erythritol (1/4 cup)

Cinnamon (1/2 teaspoon)

For the bottom layer:

Butter (2 tablespoons)

Peanut butter (4 tablespoons)

Directions

1. Set oven to 350 °F.
2. Put flaxmeal, egg white, almond flour and erythritol together in a bowl and combine.
3. Use mixture to form tart crusts in tart pans and bake for 8 minutes until crusts are set.
4. Place all ingredients for top layer of tart into a processor or blender and blend smoothly.
5. Take crusts from oven and cool. Combine ingredients for bottom layer in a microwave safe bowl and heat for 1 minute.
6. Mix together and pour into crusts, level and refrigerate for 30 minutes.
7. Top peanut butter layer with chocolate layer and smooth. Return to fridge for 30 minutes or until set.
8. Serve.

Nutritional Information

Calories 305

Net Carbs 3.9g

Fats 26.8g

Protein 9.8g

Fiber 6.6g

Honeydew & Vanilla Fat Bombs

Ingredients

1 cup coconut butter

1/2 cup fresh or honeydew

1/2 tsp sweeter to taste

1/2 tsp vanilla extract

1 Tbs lime juice

Directions

1. Place coconut butter, coconut oil and Honeydew in a pot and heat over medium heat until well combined.

2. In a small blender, add Honeydew mix and remaining ingredients. Process until smooth.

3. Spread out into a small pan lined with parchment paper. Refrigerate until mix has hardened.

4. Remove from container and cut into squares.

5. Serve.

Nutritional Information

Calories 140

Net Carbs 0,6g

Fats 15.4g

Protein 0.2g

Strawberry Ice cream

Serves 6

Ingredients

Erythritol (1/3 cup)

Vanilla (1/2 teaspoon)

Vodka (1 tablespoon)

Heavy cream (1 cup)

Egg yolks (3)

Xanthan gum (1 tablespoon)

Strawberries (1 cup, chopped into chunks)

Directions

1. Add cream to a saucepan and heat then add erythritol and stir until it dissolves. Do not boil mixture.
2. Beat egg yolks until they are twice their size. Add cream a little at a time to eggs while beating until all eggs and cream are combined; add vanilla and beat together.
3. Add xanthan gum and vodka to mixture and combine.
4. Place into a freezer safe container and freeze for 2 hours or more. You may process through an ice cream machine if you prefer.
5. Add strawberries to ice cream and mix together gently. Return to freezer for 6 hours or more.
6. Serve!

Nutritional Information

Calories 178
Net Carbs 2.8g
Fats 16.9g
Protein 2.3g
Fiber 0.5g

Strawberry Shortcake

Serves 5

Ingredients

For puff cakes:

Cream cheese (3 oz.)

Vanilla (1/2 teaspoon)

Eggs (3)

Baking powder (1/4 teaspoon)

Erythritol (2 tablespoons)

For filling:

Heavy cream (1 cup)

Strawberries (10)

Directions

1. Set oven to 300 F. Use preferred method to separate egg whites from yolks. Beat egg whites until fluffy and put aside until needed.
2. Add vanilla, erythritol, cream cheese and baking powder to egg yolks and beat together until smooth.
3. Add egg whites a little at a time to mixture and fold to combine.
4. Line a baking sheet with parchment paper or silpat and spread mixture evenly.
5. Bake for 25-30 minutes, remove from oven and cool.
6. Top with strawberries and cream, slice and serve.

Nutritional Information

Calories 178

Net Carbs 2.8g

Fats 16.9g

Protein 2.3g

Fiber 0.5g

Lemon Soufflés with Poppyseed

Serves 5

Ingredients

Eggs (2, separated)

Lemon zest (2 teaspoons)

Vanilla (1 teaspoon)

Ricotta (1 cup, whole milk)

Erythritol (1/4 cup)

Lemon juice (`1 tablespoon, freshly squeezed)

Poppy seeds (1 teaspoon)

Directions

1. Set oven to 375 F. Use preferred method to separate egg whites from yolks. Beat egg whites until fluffy and put aside until needed. Add 2 tablespoons of erythritol to egg whites and beat until egg whites become stiff.
2. Add the remaining erythritol and ricotta cheese to the egg yolks and beat until creamy.
3. Add lemon juice, poppy seeds and vanilla to egg yolk mixture. Mix together thoroughly and then add to egg whites a little at a time; fold to combine.
4. Grease ramekins and fill each with batter. Shake gently to level soufflés.
5. Bake for 20 minutes until soufflés are set with a little jiggle.
6. Cool and serve.

Nutritional Information
Calories 151
Net Carbs 2.9g
Fats 10.8g
Protein 9g
Fiber 0.1g

Mocha Ice cream

Serves 5

Ingredients

Coconut milk (1 cup)

Erythritol (2 tablespoons)

Cocoa powder (2 tablespoons)

Xanthan gum (1/4 teaspoon)

Heavy cream (1/4 cup)

Stevia (15 drops, liquid)

Instant coffee (1 tablespoon)

Directions

1. Place all ingredients into a food processor or blender excluding the gum and pulse until thoroughly combined.
2. Add gum a little at a time while processing until mixture thickens.
3. Process in an ice cream machine or freeze overnight and blend before serving.
4. Enjoy.

Nutritional Information

Calories 145

Net Carbs 1.5g

Fats 15g

Protein 1g

Fiber 2.5g

Chocolate Roll Cake

Serves 12

Ingredients

<u>For cake:</u>

Butter (4 tablespoons, melted)

Psyllium husk powder (1/4 cup)

Coconut milk (1/4 cup)

Erythritol (1/4 cup)

Baking powder (1 teaspoon)

Almond flour (1 cup)

Eggs (3)

Cocoa powder (1/4 cup)

Sour cream (1/4 cup)

Vanilla (1 teaspoon)

<u>For Filling:</u>

Butter (8 tablespoons)

Erythritol (1/4 cup)

Vanilla (1 teaspoon)

Cream cheese (8 oz.)

Sour cream (1/4 cup)

Stevia (1/4 teaspoon, liquid)

Directions

1. Set oven to 350F.

2. Put all dry ingredients for cake into a bowl and add wet ingredients one at a time and combine.

3. Line a baking sheet with parchment paper or silpat and spread cake mixture onto sheet. Try to flatten dough as much as possible

4. Bake for 12-15 minutes and cool.

5. Combine filling ingredients until smooth and spread over cake then use spatula to lift cake and roll into a log.

6. Remove excess filling from edges and slice.

7. Serve. You may chill cake before serving or until ready to serve.

Nutritional Information

Calories 274

Net Carbs 2.8g

Fat 25.1g

Protein 5.3g

Fiber 3.9g

Caramel Chocolate Brownies

Serves 8

Ingredients

Almond flour (2 cups)

Erythritol (1/3 cup)

Maple syrup (1/4 cup)

Psyllium husk powder (1 tablespoon)

Baking powder (1 teaspoon)

Cocoa powder (1/2 cup, unsweetened)

Coconut oil (1/4 cup)

Eggs (2)

Salted caramel (2 tablespoons)

Salt (1/2 teaspoon)

Directions

1. Set oven to 350F.

2. Place all wet ingredients into a bowl and mix together thoroughly.

3. Combine all dry ingredients together in a large bowl and add liquid mixture to it; mix together.

4. Grease a brownie pan and add brownie batter to pan. Bake for 20 minutes.

5. Cool, take from pan and slice.

6. Serve.

Nutritional Information

Calories 258

Net Carbs 4.5g

Fat 23.7g

Protein 8g

Fiber 5.9g

Pistachio-Almond Fat Bombs

Ingredients

1/2 cup cocoa butter, finely chopped and melted

1 cup all natural, creamy almond butter

1 cup coconut butter

1 cup coconut oil, firm

1/2 cup full fat coconut milk, chilled overnight

1/4 cup ghee

1 Tbs pure vanilla extract

2 tsp chai spice

1/4 tsp pure almond extract

1/4 tsp sea salt

1/4 cup shelled pistachios, chopped

Directions

1. Line a 9"x9" square baking pan with parchment paper, leaving a little bit hanging on either side for easy unmolding. Set aside.

2. Melt the cocoa butter in a small saucepan set over low heat or in the microwave, stirring often regardless of which option you chose. Reserve.

3. Add all ingredients, except for the cacao butter and pistachios, into a large mixing bowl. Mix with a hand mixer, starting on low speed and progressively moving to high until all the ingredients are well combined and the mixture becomes light and airy.

4. Pour the melted cacao butter right into the almond mixture and resume mixing on low speed until it's well incorporated.

5. Spread as evenly as possible into the prepared pan and sprinkle with chopped pistachios.

6. Refrigerate until completely set, at least 4 hours but preferably overnight.

7. Cut into 36 squares and store in an airtight container in the fridge.

Nutritional Information

Calories 176

Net Carbs 0.4g

Fats 18.8g

Protein 1.8g

Fiber 2.1g

Creamy Avocado Chocolate Ice cream

Serves 6

Ingredients

Hass avocados (2)

Heavy cream (1/2 cup)

Vanilla (2 teaspoons)

Stevia (25 drops, liquid)

Coconut milk (1 cup)

Cocoa powder (1/2 cup)

Erythritol (1/2 cup, powdered)

Chocolate squares (6)

Directions

1. Remove peel and pits from avocados and put into a bowl along with vanilla and coconut milk. Using an immersion blender mix until creamy. If you don't have an immersion blender you may blend in a food processor or blender.

2. Put erythritol in a grinder and pulse until fine.

3. Add ground erythritol to avocado mixture along with cocoa powder and stevia. Mix together until thoroughly combined.

4. Chop chocolate, add to mixture and transfer to a freezer safe container. Cover with plastic wrap and freeze for 12 hours or more.

5. Remove from freezer and use an immersion blender to blend smooth or process in an n ice cream maker as directed by the manufacturer.

Nutritional Information

Calories 241

Net Carbs 3.7g

Fat 22.7g

Protein 3g

Fiber 7.5g

Salted Chocolate Macadamia Balls

Ingredients

3 Tbsp Macadamia nuts

5 Tbsp cocoa powder, unsweetened

1/2 cup coconut oil

2 Tbsp Granulated Stevia (or sweetener to your choice)

coarse sea salt, to taste

Directions

1. In a saucepan mest the coconut oil. Add cocoa powder and the sweetener. Mix and remove from heat.

2. Pour cococa mixture into silicone molds until wells are 3/4 full.

3. Refrigerate in silicone molds at least 3 hours.

4. Besprinkle macadamia nuts into each well.

5. Return silicone mold to refrigerator until completely hardened.

6. Before serving, remove chocolates from silicone mold and place on a serving dish.

7. Let sit at room temperature until surface begins to glisten.

8. Enjoy!

Nutritional Information

Calories 201
Net Carbs 0.7g
Fat 22g
Protein 1.5g

Blackberry Pudding

Serves 2

Ingredients

Baking powder (1/4 teaspoon)

Coconut oil (2 tablespoons)

Heavy cream (2 tablespoons)

Lemon Zest (from 1 lemon)

Erythritol (2 tablespoons)

Coconut flour (1/4 cup)

Egg yolks (5)

Butter (2 tablespoons)

Lemon juice (2 teaspoons)

Blackberries (1/4 cup)

Stevia (10 drops, liquid)

Directions

1. Set oven to 350 F.

2. Separate egg yolks from whites and put aside until needed.

3. Place dry ingredients in a bowl and place coconut oil and butter in another bowl.

4. Beat yolks thoroughly then add stevia and erythritol and combine.

5. Sift dry mix into liquid mixture and mix together.

6. Grease ramekins and fill with batter and add 2 tablespoons blackberries to each pudding and push in batter.

7. Bake for 25 minutes, cool and serve.

Nutritional Information

Calories 477.5

Net Carbs 5.5g

Fat 43.5g

Protein 9g

Fiber 6.5g

Chunky Chocolate Cookies

Makes 16

Ingredients

Whey protein (3 tablespoons, unflavored)

Psyllium husk powder (2 tablespoons)

Vanilla extract (2 teaspoons)

Stevia (10 drops, liquid)

Egg (1)

Almond flour (1 cup)

Coconut flour (2 tablespoons)

Butter (8 tablespoons, room temperature)

Erythritol (1/4 cup)

Baking powder (1/2 teaspoon)

Chocolate (5 squares)

Directions

1. Set oven to 350 F.

2. Combine almond flour, psyllium husk, whey protein, coconut flour and baking powder together in a bowl.

3. Beat softened butter until fluffy then add stevia and erythritol and beat again.

4. Add vanilla and egg to butter mixture and mix thoroughly.

5. Add dry ingredients to wet and combine.

6. Chop chocolate and add to cookie dough and mix. Roll into a log and slice into 16 cookies.

7. Flatten each cookie and place onto a lined baking sheet.

8. Bake for 15 minutes, cool and serve.

Nutritional Information

Calories 118

Net Carbs 1.6g

Fat 10.8g

Protein 2.6g

Fiber 2.8g

Blueberry Lime Cake

Makes 2 (Serves: 10)

Ingredients

Almond flour (1 cup)

Baking powder (1 teaspoon)

Blueberry extracts (2 teaspoons)

Cream cheese (1/4 cup)

Erythritol (1/4 cup)

Lime zest

Coconut flour (2 tablespoons)

Egg whites (5)

Egg yolks (5)

Blueberries (1/4 cup)

Butter (2 tablespoons, salted)

Stevia (1/4 teaspoon, liquid)

Lime juice (from 1 lime)

Directions

1. Set oven to 325 F.

2. Combine all dry ingredients for cake in a bowl.

3. Beat yolks thoroughly then add stevia, butter, cream cheese, erythritol and blueberry extract. Mix together until smooth.

4. Add zest and lime juice to mixture and combine.

5. Add dry ingredients to wet mixture and mix thoroughly.

6. Beat egg whites and lime juice until stiff peaks form then add to cake batter. Fold together until combined.

7. Grease cake pans and pour in batter, top with blueberries and bake for 40 minutes.

8. Cool, slice and serve.

Nutritional Information

Calories 145

Net Carbs 3g

Fat 12.4g

Protein 6.4g

Fiber 1.9g

Lime Avocado Sorbet infused with Cilantro

Serves: 4

Ingredients

Hass avocados (2)

Lime zest (from 2 limes)

Lime juice (from 2 limes)

Stevia (1/4 teaspoon, liquid)

Erythritol (1/4 cup)

Coconut milk (1 cup)

Cilantro (1/2 cup, chopped)

Directions

1. Remove peel and pits from avocados and slice thinly.

2. Place avocado slices onto a piece of foil and squeeze 1/2 of a lime over avocados.

3. Place avocados into freezer for 3 hours.

4. Add coconut milk, lime zest and erythritol into a saucepan and heat over a medium flame until it comes to boil.

5. Lower heat and allow to reduce a bit (about 25%).Cool and place into a freezer friendly container and freeze until mixture gets thick.

6. Chop cilantro and add remaining lime juice.

7. Place frozen avocado and cilantro to a food processor and pulse until chunky.

8. Add stevia and coconut reduction and pulse until mixture is smooth.

Nutritional Information

Calories 180

Net Carbs 3.5g

Fat 16g

Protein 2g

Fiber 7.25g

Bacon Caramel Glazed Cake Pops

Makes 36

Ingredients

For Cake Pops:

Egg yolks (5)

Egg whites (5)

Vanilla (1/2 teaspoon)

Stevia (1/4 teaspoon, liquid)

Psyllium husk powder (2 tablespoons)

Butter (2 tablespoons)

Bacon (6 oz.)

Maple syrup (1/4 cup)

Erythritol (1/4 cup)

Almond flour (1 cup)

Baking powder (1 teaspoon)

Cream of tartar (1/2 teaspoon)

For Caramel Glaze:

Salted caramel (2 1/2 tablespoons, sugar free)

Butter (5 tablespoons)

Heavy cream (5 tablespoons)

Directions

1. Chop bacon and cook until crisp, remove from pot and place onto paper towels to remove excess oil.

2. Set oven to 325 F.

3. Add vanilla, erythritol, maple syrup and stevia to egg yolks and beat until thoroughly combined.

4. Add psyllium powder, butter, almond flour and baking powder to mixture and mix together until a thick batter is formed.

5. Clean off whisks and add tartar to whites, whisk until stiff peaks start to form.

6. Add bacon to batter along with 1/3 of egg whites and mix together. Add remaining egg whites and fold in until a wet dough if formed.

7. Grease a cake pop pan and fill with batter, close and bake for 25 minutes. Repeat with remaining batter until all is used up.

8. Take from mold and stick in lollipop sticks.

9. Prepare glaze by melting butter in a sauce pan, heat until butter gets brown then add cream and syrup.

10. Mix thoroughly and continue cooking until mixture reduces.

11. Dip pops into sauce and refrigerate for 30 minutes.

12. Serve.

Nutritional Information

Calories 80
Net Carbs 0.6g
Fat 7g
Protein 3.1g
Fiber 0.7g

Choco-cherry Donuts

Serves 8

Ingredients

Almond flour (3/4 cup)

Chocolate (3 tablespoons, chopped)

Baking powder (1 teaspoon)

Coconut oil (2 ½ tablespoons)

Dark chocolate (5 bars, chopped)

Flaxmeal (1/4 cup)

Vanilla (1 teaspoon)

Eggs (2)

Coconut milk (3 tablespoons)

Berry extract (2 teaspoons)- you may choose your preferred flavor

Directions

1. Combine all dry ingredients in a large bowl; in another bowl combine all wet ingredients.
2. Add wet ingredients to dry and mix together thoroughly.
3. Add chopped dark chocolate to batter and fold.
4. Heat donut maker and grease then pipe batter into molds. If you don't have a donut maker you may use a donut pan and bake donuts for 10 minutes at 300 F.
5. Cook donuts for about 5 minutes until done.
6. Cool and serve.

Nutritional Information

Calories 107
Net Carbs 1.3g
Fats 9.4g
Protein 3.1g
Fiber 4.8g

Maple Pecan Bacon covered in Chocolate

Makes 13

Ingredients

Bacon (13 slices)

Maple extract (1 tablespoon)

Erythritol (2 tablespoons)

For coating:

Pecans (1/4 cup, chopped

Erythritol (2 tablespoons)

Cocoa powder (4 tablespoons, unsweetened)

Stevia (15 drops, liquid)

Directions

1. Set oven to 400 F.
2. Line a baking sheet with foil and spread bacon on sheet. Coat bacon with maple extract and erythritol all over.
3. Bake for 40 minutes until bacon is crisp and golden.
4. Pour excess bacon grease into a container. Add stevia, cocoa powder and erythritol to grease and stir until combined.
5. Dip bacon slices into mixture and coat with pecans.
6. Cool bacon slices and refrigerate.
7. Serve.

Nutritional Information

Calories 157
Net Carbs 0.4g
Fats 11.7g
Protein 10.5g
Fiber 0.8g

Peanut butter and Chocolate Mug Cake

Serves 1

Ingredients

Egg (1)

Almond flour (2 tablespoons)

Stevia (7 drops)

Vanilla (1/2 teaspoon)

Peanut butter (1 tablespoon)

Butter (2 tablespoons)

Erythritol (1 tablespoon)

Baking powder (1/2 teaspoon)

Dark chocolate (1 bar, chopped)

Directions

1. Combine all ingredients in a mug.
2. Place in microwave for 2 minutes.
3. Take from microwave and cool.
4. Serve. May be topped with cream.

Nutritional Information

Calories 488
Net Carbs 5g
Fats 47g
Protein 13g
Fiber 6g

Vanilla Latte Cookie

Makes 10

Ingredients

Almond flour (1 ½ cups)

Erythritol (1/3 cup)

Instant coffee (1 tablespoon + 1 teaspoon))

Baking soda (1/2 teaspoon)

Cinnamon (1/4 teaspoon)

Butter (1/2 cup, unsalted)

Eggs (2)

Vanilla (1 ½ teaspoons)

Kosher salt (1/2 teaspoon)

Stevia (17 drops)

Directions

1. Set oven to 350 F.
2. Combine coffee, salt, cinnamon, almond flour and baking soda in a large mixing bowl.
3. Separate egg yolks from whites in another container.
4. Put butter into a bowl and beat until slightly fluffy then add erythritol and beat until pale. Put in yolks and continue beating until mixture is smooth.
5. Add half of flour mixture to butter and combine then add stevia, vanilla and leftover flour mixture. Combine thoroughly.
6. Beat egg whites until fluffy and stiff peaks start to form. Add to batter and fold.
7. Spoon mixture onto a lined baking sheet and bake for 15 minutes.
8. Cool and serve.

Nutritional Information

Calories 167

Net Carbs 1.4g

Fats 17.1g

Protein 3.9g

Fiber 14g

Almond Butter and Chia Seeds Bars

Makes 14

Ingredients

Coconut oil (1 tablespoon and 1 teaspoon)

Butter (2 tablespoons)

Stevia (1/4 teaspoon, liquid)

Coconut flakes (1/2 cup, shredded and unsweetened)

Coconut cream (1/2 cup)

Almonds (1/2 cup)

Erythritol (4 tablespoons)

Heavy cream (1/4 cup)

Vanilla (1 1/2 teaspoons)

Chia seeds (1/4 cup)

Coconut flour (2 tablespoons)

Directions

1. Place almonds in a processor and grind finely then add 2 tablespoons erythritol and 1 teaspoon of coconut oil. Mix until thoroughly combined.
2. Heat butter in a saucepan until browned and put in remaining erythritol, vanilla, stevia and cream. Stir to combine and heat until mixture starts to bubble. Add almond mixture to pot and mix together.
3. Put chia seeds into a grinder and pulse until fine and combine with coconut flakes in a pan. Heat pan and toast for a couple of minutes.
4. Combine all ingredients along with cream, coconut flour and oil. Pour into a square pan and put into fridge for 60 minutes.
5. Slice into bars and keep chilled until ready to serve.

Nutritional Information
Calories 120

Net Carbs 1.4g

Fats 11.1g

Protein 2.4g

Fiber 2.6g

Lemon Sponge Cake

Makes 3

Ingredients

For Cake:
Baking powder (1 teaspoon)
Egg yolks (5)
Egg whites (5)
Almond extract (1 teaspoon)
Liquid stevia (1/4 teaspoon)
Olive oil (2 tablespoons)
Almond flour (1 cup)
Salt (1/4 teaspoon)
Vanilla (1 teaspoon)
Erythritol (1/4 cup)
Lemon zest (from 1/2 lemon)
Cream of tartar (1/2 teaspoon)

For Raspberry Icing:
Heavy cream (4 tablespoons)
Lemon juice (from 1/2 of a lemon)
Butter (4 tablespoons)
Raspberries (1/3 cup)

Directions
1. Set oven to 325 F.
2. Combine all dry ingredients except tartar and in another bowl mix together all wet ingredients except zest and egg whites.
3. Add tartar to egg whites and beat until stiff peaks form.

4. Add egg white mix to cake batter and fold until thoroughly combined.

5. Grease cake pan and pour in batter; bake for 25 minutes.

6. Prepare icing by heating butter until golden then add lemon juice and cream, whisk and remove from heat.

7. Add raspberries and use spoon to crush as you combine mixture. Cool for 15 minutes.

8. Pour on top of cakes before serving.

9. Serve and enjoy.

Nutritional Information

Calories 414

Net Carbs 7.1g

Fats 38g

Protein 18g

Fiber 9.6g

Coffee Cake

Serves 8

Ingredients

For Cake:
Cream cheese (6 oz.)
Liquid stevia (1/4 teaspoon)
Vanilla extract (2 teaspoons)
Egg yolks (6)
Egg whites (6)
Erythritol (1/4 cup)
Protein powder (1/4 cup, unflavored)
Cream of tartar (1/4 teaspoon)

For filling:
Almond flour (1 1/2 cups)
Butter (1/2 stick)
Erythritol (1/4 cup)
Cinnamon (1 tablespoon)
Maple syrup (1/4 cup)

Directions
1. Set oven to 325 °F.
2. Add egg yolks to erythritol and beat together then add all ingredients except egg white and tartar. Mix together to combine.
3. Combine tartar and white until peaks form.
4. Add half of egg whites to batter and fold in then add the remainder of egg whites and fold again.

5. Combine all filling ingredients until dough like mixture if formed.

6. Add cake mixture to pan and top with as much of filling mixture as you can.

7. Bake for 20 minutes and top with leftover filling.

8. Bake for 20 minutes more, cool and serve.

Nutritional Information
Calories 257

Net Carbs 3.8g

Fats 26.7g

Protein 12.8g

Fiber 2.2g

Chocolate Dipped Macaroons

Makes 12

Ingredients

Coconut (1 cup, unsweetened and shredded)

Erythritol (1/4 cup)

Salt

Coconut oil (2 tablespoons)

Egg white (1)

Almond extract (1/2 teaspoon)

Chocolate (20 grams, sugar free)

Directions

1. Set oven to 350 F.
2. Line baking sheet with parchment paper and spread shredded coconut onto sheet; toast in oven for 5 minutes.
3. Beat the egg whites then add salt, almond extract and erythritol and beat again to combine.
4. Remove coconut from oven, cool and add to egg mixture.
5. Using a spoon or scoop, drop macaroons onto a lined baking sheet and bake for 15 minutes until golden.
6. Heat coconut oil until it melts in a saucepan then add chocolate and cook until it melts. Stir to avoid burning.
7. Dip macaroons into chocolate mixture and return to baking sheet to cool.
8. Serve.

Nutritional Facts

Calories 73

Net Carbs 1g

Fats 7.3g

Protein 1g

Fiber 1.7g

Spiced Lemon Glazed Fritters

Serves 6

Ingredients

Erythritol (3 tablespoons)

Egg (1)

Cinnamon (1/2 teaspoon)

Lemon zest (from 1/2 of lemon)

Almond flour (1/2 cup)

Baking powder (1 teaspoon)

Xanthan gum (1/2 teaspoon)

Vanilla (1/2 teaspoon)

Fat of choice (2 cups)

<u>For glaze:</u>

Erythritol (3 tablespoons, powder)

Lemon juice from 1/2 of lemon

Directions

1. Put all dry ingredients for fritter into a bowl and mix together.

2. Add egg to dry mix and combine to form a sticky dough.

3. Heat oil in a deep pot and use spoon to drop fritters into hot oil. Fry fritters until golden.

4. Combine ingredients for glaze until smooth and use to top fritters

5. Cool and serve.

Nutritional Facts

Calories 50

Net Carbs 0.7g

Fats 4.6g

Protein 1.7g

Fiber 7g

Cinnamon Bun Balls

Serves 8

Ingredients

1 cup coconut butter

1 cup full fat coconut milk (from a can)

1 cup unsweetened coconut shreds

1 tsp vanilla extract

1/2 tsp cinnamon

1/2 tsp nutmeg

1 tsp sugar substitute such as Splenda

Directions

1. Combine all ingredients except the shredded coconut together in double boiler or a bowl set over a pan of simmering water. Stir until everything is melted and combined.

2. Remove bowl from heat and place in the fridge until the mixture has firmed up and can be rolled into balls.

3. Form the mixture into 1" balls, a small cookie scoop is helpful for doing this.

4. Roll each ball in the shredded coconut until well coated.

5. Serve and enjoy! Store in the fridge.

Nutritional Facts

Calories 42

Net Carbs 0.6g

Fats 4.6g

Protein 0.7g

Fiber 1g

Raspberry Cheesecake Cups

Serves 12

Ingredients

Almond meal (1/2 cup)

Stevia (1/2 cup)

Eggs (2)

Butter (4 tablespoons, melted)

Cream cheese (16 oz., softened)

Vanilla (1 teaspoon)

Raspberry syrup (1/4 cup, sugarfree)

Directions

1. Set oven to 350 F and line baking molds.

2. Combine almond meal with melted butter and put into molds.

3. Add eggs, syrup, vanilla, cream cheese and Stevia to a bowl and use a hand mixer to cream mixture.

4. Use mixture to fill molds and bake for 15 minutes.

5. Remove from oven, cool for 10 minutes and refrigerate for 30 minutes.

6. Serve.

Nutritional Facts

Calories 206

Net Carbs 2.1g

Fats 19g

Protein 5g

Fiber 6g

Chocolate filled Fried Cookie Dough

Serves 12

Ingredients

Almond flour (3/4 cup)

Eggs (2)

Coconut oil (2 tablespoons)

Chocolate (3 squares)

Erythritol (1 teaspoon, powdered)

Casein powder (1 scoop, vanilla)

Stevia (10 drops)

Baking powder (1/2 tablespoon)

Granulated erythritol (2 teaspoons)

Directions

1. Combine almond flour, casein powder and baking powder.

2. Add granulated erythritol, stevia and egg to mixture and mix to combine until dough forms.

3. Form dough into a rectangular shape and slice into 12 pieces.

4. Chop each chocolate square into four parts. Take each slice of dough and make a well in the center of each.

5. Seal and roll into balls then heat oil in a frying pan.

6. Cook cookie balls until golden all over. Remove from pot, place on paper towels to remove excess oil.

7. Sprinkle with left over erythritol as they cool.

8. Serve.

Nutritional Facts

Calories 88

Net Carbs 1.9g

Fats 7.2g

Protein 4.7g

Fiber 12.8g

Coconut and Macadamia Custard

Makes 4

Ingredients

Eggs (4)

Macadamia Butter (1/3 cup)

Liquid stevia (1 teaspoon)

Coconut milk (1 cup, unsweetened)

Heavy cream (1/3 cup)

Vanilla (1 teaspoon)

Erythritol (1/3 cup)

Directions

1. Set oven to 325 F.
2. Place all ingredients into a bowl and whisk together to combine. Be sure not to overmix the batter.
3. Add an inch of water to a baking pan and place ramekins into water. Divide batter equally amongst ramekins and bake for 40 minutes.
4. Cool for 45 minutes and place in refrigerator until ready to serve.

Nutritional Facts

Calories 88
Net Carbs 1.9g
Fats 7.2g
Protein 4.7g
Fiber 6.3g

Choco- peanut butter Ice cream

Serves 6

Ingredients

Almond milk (1/2 cup)

Egg yolks (3)

Xanthan gum (1/4 teaspoon)

Chocolate chips (3/4 cup, sugar-free)

Heavy cream (1/2 cup)

Erythritol (1/4 cup)

Vanilla (1 teaspoon)

Vodka (1 tablespoon)

Peanut butter (1/2 cup)

Directions

1. Add erythritol and cream to a saucepan and heat over a low flame until it starts to simmer.
2. Whisk vanilla and yolks together and add heated mixture a little at a time to eggs while whisking.
3. Return mixture to saucepan over a low flame and add gum to mixture, whisk until mixture thickens slightly.
4. Strain mixture through a fine sieve and add vodka. Refrigerate until chilled.
5. Process through an ice-cream machine according to the instructions.
6. Add peanut butter in the final second and freeze until ready to serve.
7. Enjoy.

Nutritional Facts

Calories 295

Net Carbs 5.8g

Fats 26g

Protein 8g

Fiber 2g

Jelly cookies

Makes 16

Ingredients

Coconut flour (2 tablespoons)

Cinnamon (1/4 teaspoon)

Erythritol (1/2 cup)

Coconut oil (4 tablespoons)

Almond extract (1/2 teaspoon)

Coconut (1 tablespoon, shredded)

Almond flour (1 cup)

Baking powder (1/2 teaspoon)

Salt (1/2 teaspoon)

Eggs (2)

Vanilla extract (1/2 teaspoon)

Jam of choice (2 tablespoons, sugar-free)

Directions

1. Set oven to 350 F.

2. Place all dry ingredients in a bowl and whisk together to combine. Combine wet ingredients and add to dry mix. Mix together until thoroughly combined.

3. Line a baking sheet with parchment paper and shape cookies on sheet. Make an indent in the center of each cookie.

4. Bake for 16 minutes until golden, remove from oven and cool.

5. Fill each indent with jam and coconut.

6. Serve.

Nutritional Facts

Calories 86

Net Carbs 1.2g

Fats 7.9g

Protein 2.4g

Fiber 1.3g

Peanut Butter Truffles

Makes 12

Ingredients

Peanut butter (1 cup)

Erythritol (1 ½ cups, powdered)

Butter (4 tablespoons, melted)

Chocolate (6 oz., sugar-free)

Directions

1. Combine erythritol, butter and peanut butter in a bowl until mixture binds together.
2. Roll batter into balls and place on a lined baking sheet. Refrigerate for 30 minutes or until very cold.
3. Melt chocolate in a saucepan and check consistency, should be thick enough to stick to truffles.
4. Use a spoon to dip truffles into melted chocolate, coat all sides of truffles.
5. Refrigerate to set and serve.

Nutritional Facts

Calories 200
Net Carbs 5g
Fats 17g
Protein 5.9g
Fiber 3g

Lava Cake

Makes 1

Ingredients

Erythritol (2 tablespoons)

Heavy cream (1 tablespoon)

Baking powder (1/4teaspoon)

Cocoa powder (2 tablespoons)

Egg (1)

Vanilla (1/2 teaspoon)

Salt

Directions

1. Set oven to 350 F.
2. Combine cocoa powder with erythritol in a bowl and in another bowl whisk egg until fluffy.
3. Add vanilla, cream, baking powder, salt and egg to cocoa mix.
4. Grease a ramekin and add batter to it; bake for 14 minutes. Do not bake too much; cake should not be too firm. Serve.

Nutritional Facts

Calories 173
Net Carbs 4g
Fats 13g
Protein 8g
Fiber 5g

Creamy Pistachio Strawberry Popsicles

Makes 4

Ingredients

Pistachios (2 oz., salted)

Almond milk (1/2 cup)

Strawberries (8 oz.)

Heavy cream (1/2 cup)

Stevia (15 drops)

Directions

1. Put strawberries in a processor along with milk, stevia and cream. Pulse until all ingredients are combined.
2. Add pistachios and fold in; do not blend.
3. Pour mixture into popsicle molds and freeze for 3 hours or more.
4. Serve.

Nutritional Facts

Calories 158
Net Carbs 5.6g
Fats 12.5g
Protein 4g
Fiber 3g

Lemony Cheesecake Mousse

Serves 5

Ingredients

Lemon juice (1/4 cup)

Lemon stevia (1 teaspoon, liquid)

Mascarpone cheese (8 oz.)

Salt (1/8 teaspoon)

Heavy cream (1 cup)

Directions

1. Add lemon juice and cheese to a bowl and use a hand mixer to combine until smooth.
2. Add lemon juice, salt and cream to mixture and whip until fluffy.
3. Pipe mixture into glasses and top with zest.
4. Chill and serve.

Nutritional Facts

Calories 277
Net Carbs 1.7g
Fats 29.6g
Protein 3.7g
Fiber 0g

Macchiato Cheesecake

Serves 9

Ingredients

For Cheesecake Base

Butter (2 tablespoons, unsalted)

Caramel syrup (1 tablespoon, sugar-free)

Cream cheese (8 oz., soft)

Espresso concentrate (3 tablespoons, cold)

Stevia (1/3 cup)

For frosting:

Caramel syrup (3 tablespoons, sugar free)
Mascarpone cheese (8 oz., soft)
Butter (3 tablespoons, unsalted, softened)
Splenda (2 tablespoons)

Directions

1. Set oven to 350°F.

2. Place all ingredients for cheesecake in a bowl and use a mixer to blend together until smooth.

3. Grease cupcake pan and add batter; bake for 15 minutes.

4. Take from oven, cool and refrigerate for 3 hours or more.

5. Prepare frosting by add all ingredients to a bowl and using a mixer to cream. Be sure to cream on low speed.

6. Top cakes with frosting and serve.

Nutritional Facts

Calories 286
Net Carbs 1g
Fats 29g
Protein 5g
Fiber 3g

Lemon and Blackberry Mini Tarts

Makes 10

Ingredients

For crust:

Egg (1)

Coconut (3/4 cup, shredded)

Macadamia nuts (1 cup)

For filling:

Lemon juice from ½ lemon
Erythritol (1/4 cup)
Gelatin powder (1 ½ tablespoons)
Coconut milk (1 cup)
Lemon zest (1 tablespoon)
Stevia (15 drops)
Water (3 tablespoons)

For Topping:

Blackberries (1 cup)

Directions

1. Set oven to 400 F.

2. Add coconut milk to a saucepan along with stevia, erythritol and lemon zest. Stir together, heat but do not boil and take from heat.

3. Combine gelatin with water and add to mixture in pot. Mix together until thoroughly combined; put aside to cool and thicken.

4. Crush nuts in a processor to desired consistency and then add to a bowl. Pulse coconut and add to nuts then add egg and mix together until mixture binds together.

5. Line a cupcake tin with paper liners and press base into each mold. Bake for 7 minutes and take from oven.

6. Top with filling and blackberries and refrigerate for 30 minutes or more.

7. Serve

Nutritional Facts

Calories 178

Net Carbs 2.8g

Fats 16.2g

Protein 4.4g

Fiber 3.1g

Lemon Soufflés

Makes 4

Ingredients

Eggs (2)

Lemon zest (2 teaspoons)

Vanilla (1 teaspoon)

Ricotta (1 cup, whole milk)

Erythritol (1/4 cup)

Lemon juice (1 tablespoon, fresh)

Poppy seeds (1 teaspoon)

Directions

1. Set oven to 375 F.

2. Separate eggs and add 2 tablespoons erythritol to whites and beat until stiff peaks start to form.

3. Add remaining erythritol to egg yolks along with ricotta cheese and beat until mixture is creamy.

4. Add lemon juice and zest to cheese mixture, stir and add poppy seeds and vanilla.

5. Add egg whites a little at a time to ricotta mixture and fold to combine.

6. Grease ramekins and fill with soufflé mixture. Shake containers to level the soufflés.

7. Bake for 20 minutes.

8. Serve.

Nutritional Facts

Calories 151

Net Carbs 2.9g

Fats 10.8g

Protein 9g

Fiber 0g

Caramel Pots

Serves 4

Ingredients

Heavy cream (1 ½ cups)

Liquid stevia (1/4 teaspoon)

Egg yolks (4)

Maple syrup (1 tablespoon)

Maple extract (1 teaspoon)

Erythritol (1/4 cup, powdered)

Salt (1/4 teaspoon)

Water (6 tablespoons)

Vanilla extract (1/2 teaspoon)

Directions

1. Set oven to 300 °F.

2. Combine water and erythritol in a saucepan and heat until mixture starts to boil. Add maple syrup and mix together. Boil for 3 minutes until mixture reduces and is syrupy.

3. Add cream, maple extract, sat, stevia and vanilla to another saucepan. Bring to a boil then lower heat and add erythritol mixture slowly while stirring.

4. Add mixture a little at a time to egg yolks and mix thoroughly. You may strain the mixture if you choose to.

5. Fill a baking pan large enough to hold your ramekins with about an inch of water. Place ramekins into pan and add mixture to ramekins.

6. Bake for 40 minutes.

7. Serve warm or cold.

Nutritional Facts

Calories 359

Net Carbs 3g

Fats 34.9g

Protein 2.8g

Fiber 0g

Whisky Vanilla Mug Cake

Serves 1-2

Ingredients

Egg (1)

Almond flour (3 tablespoons)

Stevia (7 drops)

Whisky (1 tablespoon)

Coconut flour (2 teaspoons)

Butter (2 tablespoons)

Erythritol (1 tablespoon)

Baking powder (1/2 teaspoon)

Vanilla (1/2 teaspoon)

Directions

1. Combine all ingredients in a microwave safe mug until thoroughly combined.

2. Place in microwave for 2 minutes.

3. Serve in mug or turn upside down and remove from mug onto a plate.

4. Enjoy.

Nutritional Facts

Calories 448

Net Carbs 5g

Fats 40g

Protein 12g

Fiber 4g

Maple Pecan Muffins

Serves 5

Ingredients

Flaxseed (1/2 cup)

Coconut oil (1/2 cup)

Erythritol (1/4 cup)

Vanilla extract (1 teaspoon)

Apple cider vinegar (1/2 teaspoon)

Almond flour (1 cup)

Pecans (3/4 cup)

Eggs (2)

Maple extract (2 teaspoons)

Baking soda (1/2 teaspoon)

Stevia (1/4 teaspoon, liquid)

Directions

1. Set oven to 325 F.

2. Put pecan in a processor and pulse until chopped. Transfer to a large bowl reserving 1/3 of pecans until needed.

3. Add remaining dry ingredients to pecans and combine liquids together in another bowl. Add wet ingredients to dry mix and combine.

4. Line cupcake pan/muffin tin and add batter then top with reserved pecans.

5. Bake for 30 minutes, remove and cool.

6. Serve.

Nutritional Facts

Calories 208

Net Carbs 1.5g

Fats 20.7g

Protein 4.8g

Fiber 2.8g

Chocolate Blackberry Panna Cotta

Serves 10

Ingredients

Cream cheese (12 oz.)

Butter (3 tablespoons)

Erythritol (2 tablespoons)

Gelatin powder (2 ½ teaspoons)

Water (1 cup)

Blackberry preserves (3 tablespoons +1 teaspoon)

Cocoa powder (3 tablespoons)

Vanilla (1 teaspoon)

Liquid stevia (10 drops)

Directions

1. Place softened butter, vanilla and cream cheese in a bowl and use mixer to cream mixture.

2. Heat water and combine with erythritol and gelatin then add to cream cheese mixture.

3. Carefully blend mixture until creamy and smooth then add cocoa and blend again.

4. Grease cupcake molds and pour in batter; place in fridge for 20 minutes.

5. Divide preserves amongst panna cotta and stir to combine. Return to fridge and set overnight.

6. Serve.

Nutritional Facts

Calories 156.2

Net Carbs 24.5g

Fats 15.8g

Protein 2.9g

Fiber 1.6g

Snickerdoodle Cookies

Makes 14

Ingredients

For cookies:

Coconut oil (1/4 cup)

Vanilla (1 tablespoon)

Liquid Stevia (7 drops)

Macadamia nuts (1/3 cup)

Almond flour (2 cups)

Maple syrup (1/4 cup)

Baking soda (1/4 teaspoon)

Salt

For topping:

Erythritol (2 tablespoons)
Cinnamon (2 tablespoons)

Directions

1. Set oven to 350 F.

2. Combine salt, baking soda and flour in a large bowl.

3. In another container combine maple syrup, stevia, oil and vanilla. Crush nuts in a processor.

4. Add wet ingredients to dry and mix together. Combine ingredients for topping in another container.

5. Form dough into balls, roll in toppings mixture and place on a lined baking sheet.

6. Flatten and bake cookies for 10 minutes.

7. Cool and serve.

Nutritional Facts

Calories 155

Net Carbs 2.1g

Fats 14.8g

Protein 3.6g

Fiber 2.5g

Chocolate Almond Cookies

Servings: 12

Ingredients

2 cups almond meal

1 1/2 tsp almond extract

4 Tbsp cocoa powder

5 Tbsp coconut oil, melted

2 Tbsp almond milk

4 Tbsp agave nectar

2 tsp vanilla extract

1/8 tsp baking soda

1/8 tsp salt

Directions

1. Preheat oven to 340F degrees.
2. In a deep bowl mix salt, cocoa powder, almond meal and baking soda.
3. In a separate bowl, whisk together melted coconut oil, almond milk, almond and vanilla extract and maple syrup. Merge the almond meal mixture with almond milk mixture and mix well.
4. In a greased baking pan pour the batter evenly. Bake for 10-15 minutes. 5. Once ready let cool on a wire rack and serve.

Nutritional Facts

Calories 79.32g

Net Carbs 2.1g

Fats 5.94g

Protein 0.46g

Fiber 0.61g

Lemon & Coconut Balls

Serves 4

Ingredients

3 packages of True Lemon (Crystallized Citrus for Water)

1/4 cup shredded coconut, unsweetened

1 cup cream cheese

1/4 cup granulated Stevia

Directions

1. In a bowl, combine cream cheese, lemon and Stevia. Blend well until incorporate.
2. Once the mixture is well combined, put it back in the fridge to harden up a bit.
3. Roll into 16 balls and dip each ball into shredded coconut. Refrigerate for several hours. Serve.

Nutritional Facts

Calories 216

Net Carbs 3.12g

Fats 21.50g

Protein 3.61g

Fiber 0.45g

Chocolate Chia Cream

Serves 4

Ingredients

1/4 cup Chia seeds

1 cup heavy whipping cream

1 cup coconut milk

2 Tbs cocoa powder

pure vanilla extract

1/4 cup Erythritol sweetener

Directions

1. In a bowl mix the chia seeds and add the coconut milk until it combines well.
2. Add the Erythritol and whisk some more. Divide the mixture into two portions.
3. Add cocoa to one half and mixed it nicely.
4. Pour chia seed mixture into the bowls or glasses. Keep covered in the refrigerator for 12 hours.
5. Before serving beat the heavy whipping cream and pour over the chia seeds cream. Enjoy!

Nutritional Facts
Calories 341,31
Net Carbs 7.35g
Fats 35.41g
Protein 2.99g
Fiber 1.56g

Peanut Butter Delights

Serves: 16

Ingredients

2 eggs

2 1/2 cup of peanut butter

1/2 cup shredded coconut (unsweetened)

1/2 cup of Xylitol

1 Tbsp of pure vanilla extract

Directions

1. Preheat oven to 320 F.
2. Mix all ingredients together by your hands.
3. After the ingredients are thoroughly mixed, roll into heaped tablespoon sized balls and press into a baking tray lined with baking paper.
4. Bake in the oven for 12 minutes or until the tops of the cookies are browning. When ready, let cool on a wire rack. Ready!
1. Serve.

Nutritional Facts

Calories 254
Net Carbs 8.31g
Fats 21.75g
Protein 10.98g
Fiber 2.64g

Watermelon Soup

Serves 1

Ingredients

Watermelon (3/4 cups, seeds removed)

Sour cream (2 tablespoons)

Lemon juice (1/4 teaspoon)

Heavy cream (1/2 cup, whipped)

Raspberries (1/4 cup)

Vanilla Stevia (1 tablespoon)

Mint (1/4 teaspoon, fresh, chopped)

Directions

1. Add all ingredients except whipped cream to a blender and pulse until thoroughly combined.

2. Pour into a bowl and top with cream.

3. Serve.

Nutritional Facts

Calories 192
Net Carbs 8g
Fats 17g
Protein 2g
Fiber 1g

Vanilla & Lime Cheesecake

Serves 2

Ingredients

1/4 cup cream cheese, softened

2 Tbsp heavy cream

1 tsp lime juice

1 egg

1 tsp pure vanilla extract

2-4 Tbsp Eerythritol or Stevia

Directions

1. In a microwave-safe bowl combine all ingredients. Place in a microwave and cook on HIGH for 90 seconds.

2. Every 30 seconds stir to combine the ingredients well.

3. Transfer mixture to a bowl and refrigerate for at least 2 hours.

4. Before serving top with whipped cream or coconut powder.

Nutritional Facts

Calories 140
Net Carbs 1.38g
Fats 13.04g
Protein 4.34g
Fiber 0.02g

English Toffee Balls

Serves: 24

Ingredients

1 cup coconut oil

2 Tbsp butter

1/2 block cream cheese, softened

3/4 Tbsp cocoa powder

1/2 cup creamy, natural peanut butter

3 Tbsp Davinci Gourmet Sugar Free English Toffee Syrup

Directions

1. Combine all ingredients in a saucepan over medium heat.

2. Stir until everything is smooth, melted, and combined.

3. Pour mixture into small candy molds or mini muffin tins lined with paper liners.

4. Freeze or refrigerate until set and enjoy!

5. Store in an airtight container in the fridge.

Nutritional Facts

Calories 136
Net Carbs 0.3g
Fats 15g
Protein 1.7g
Fiber 0.04g

Fresh Choc-Mint Fat Bombs

Serves 6

Ingredients

1/2 cup coconut oil melted

2 Tbsp cocoa powder

1 Tbsp granulated stevia, or sweetener of choice, to taste

2 Tbsp mint leaves (fresh, finely chopped)

Directions

1. Mix the melted coconut oil with the finely chopped peppermint leaves and sweetener.

2. Pour half the mixture into silicon cases or ice cube trays. Place in the fridge. This will become the white layer.

3. Add the cocoa powder to the remaining mixture, then pour onto the white layer which has set in the fridge.

4. Keep refrigerated until set completely.

Nutritional Facts

Calories 161
Net Carbs 0.3g
Fats 18,5g
Protein 0.4g
Fiber 0.07g

Chocolate & Almond Biscotti

Serves 8

Ingredients

1 egg

2 cups whole almonds

2 Tbs flax seeds

1 cup shredded coconut, unsweetened

1 cup coconut oil

1 cup cacao powder

1/4 cup Xilitol or Stevia sweetener

1 tsp salt

1 tsp baking soda

Directions

1. Preheat oven to 350F.
2. In a food process blend the whole almonds with the flax seeds. Add in the rest of ingredients and mix well.
3. Place the dough on a piece of aluminum foil to shape into 8 biscotti-shaped slices. Bake for 12 minutes.
4. Let cool and serve.

Nutritional Facts

Calories 276,56
Net Carbs 9.19g
Fats 25,44g
Protein 8,24g
Fiber 5.2g

Pumpkin Spice Blondies

Serves 12

Ingredients

Butter (1/2 cup, softened)

Egg (1)

Cinnamon (1 teaspoon)

Maple extract (1 teaspoon)

Almond flour (1/4 cup)

Pecans (1 oz., chopped)

Erythritol (1/2 cup)

Liquid Stevia (15 drops)

Pumpkin puree (1/2 cup)

Pumpkin pie spice (1/8 teaspoon)

Coconut flour (2 tablespoons)

Directions

1. Set oven to 350 F.

2. Add butter, egg, pumpkin puree and erythritol to a bowl and beat with a hand mixer until smooth.

3. Add coconut flour, stevia, maple extract, almond flour, cinnamon and pumpkin spice to mixture and mix together.

4.   Grease brownie pan and pour in batter.

5.   Top mixture with pecans and bake for 25 minutes until golden.

6.   Take from oven, cool and slice.

7.   Serve.

Nutritional Facts

Calories 112

Net Carbs 1.4g

Fats 10.8g

Protein 1.4g

Fiber 1.3g

Peanut-Butter Cookie Balls

Serves 18

Ingredients

2 cups peanut butter

1/4 cup Erythritol

2 eggs

1 1/4 cups coconut flour

2 tsp baking soda

2 tsp peanut extract

1/2 tsp kosher salt

Directions

1. Preheat oven to 345° F.
2. In a bowl beat the peanut butter, coconut flour and Erythritol with an electric mixer (MEDIUM speed) until fluffy.
3. Reduce speed to LOW and add in the eggs, baking soda, vanilla, and salt.
4. With your hands make balls from the batter and place on parchment-lined baking pan. Bake 10 to 15 minutes.
5. When ready, cool slightly and then move from the stove to cool completely.
6. Serve.

Nutritional Facts
Calories 182,5
Net Carbs 1.4g
Fats 14,67g
Protein 7g
Fiber 1.96g

Delicious Nuts Bars

Serves 10

Ingredients

1 cup almonds

1/2 cup hazelnut, chopped

1 cup peanuts

1 cup shredded coconut

1 cup almond butter

1 cup Liquid Erythritol

1 cup coconut oil, freshly melted and still warm

Directions

1. In a food processor place all nuts and chop for 1-2 minutes.
2. Add in grated coconut, almond butter, Erythritol and coconut oil. Process it for 1 minute about.
3. Cover a square bowl with parchment paper and place the mixture on top.
4. Flatten the mixture with a spatula. Place the bowl in the freezer for 4-5 hours.
5. Remove batter from the freezer, cut and serve.

Nutritional Facts
Calories 193,62
Net Carbs 5.4g
Fats 18,2g
Protein 3.38g
Fiber 2.53g

Sticky Chocolate Fudge Squares

Serves 12

Ingredients

1 cup coconut oil, softened

1/4 cup coconut milk (full fat, from a can)

1/4 cup cocoa powder

1 teaspoon vanilla extract

1/2 teaspoon sea salt

1-3 drops liquid stevia

Directions

1. With a hand mixer or stand mixer, whip the softened coconut oil and coconut milk together until smooth and glossy. About 6 minutes on high.

2. Add the cocoa powder, vanilla extract, sea salt, and one drop of liquid stevia to the bowl and mix on low until combined. Increase speed once everything is combined and mix for one minute. Taste fudge and adjust sweetness by adding additional liquid stevia, if desired.

3. Prepare a 9"x4" loaf pan by lining it with parchment paper.

4. Pour fudge into loaf pan and place in freezer for about 15, until just set.

5. Remove fudge and cut into 1" x 1" pieces. Store in an airtight container in the fridge or freezer.

Nutritional Facts

Calories 172

Net Carbs 5.4g

Fats 19,6g

Protein 3.38g

Fiber 2.53g

Coco - Raspberry Fat Bombs

Serves 12

Ingredients

1/2 cup coconut butter

1/2 cup coconut oil

1/2 cup freeze dried raspberries

1/2 cup unsweetened shredded coconut

1/4 powdered sugar substitute such as Swerve or Truvia

Directions

1. Line an 8"x8" pan with parchment paper.

2. In a food processor, coffee grinder, or blender, pulse the dried raspberries into a fine powder.

3. In a saucepan over medium heat, combine the coconut butter, coconut oil, coconut, and sweetener. Stir until melted and well combined.

4. Remove pan from heat and stir in raspberry powder.

5. Pour mixture into pan and refrigerate or freeze for several hours, or overnight.

6. Cut into 12 pieces and serve!

Nutritional Facts
Calories 234
Net Carbs 1.1g
Fats 23.6g
Protein 3.9g
Fiber 3.8g

Blueberry Power Fat Bombs

Serves 6

Ingredients

5 Tbsp butter

3 Tbsp coconut oil

2 Tbsp sugar-free Blueberry syrup

2 Tbsp cocoa powder

Directions

1. In a sauce pan add all ingredients and cook over low heat until chocolate sauce texture.
2. Pour into mold and freeze for at least 3 hours.
3. Before serving unmold and enjoy.

Nutritional Facts

Calories 148

Net Carbs 0.05g

Fats 17g

Protein 0.5g

Fiber 0.6g

Chia and Pecan Butter Blondies

Makes 16

Ingredients

Pecans (2 ¼ cups, roasted)

Butter (1/4 cup, melted)

Salted caramel (3 tablespoons, sugar free)

Eggs (3)

Heavy cream (3 tablespoons)

Chia seeds (1/2 cup, ground)

Erythritol (1/4 cup, powdered)

Liquid stevia (10 drops)

Baking powder (1 teaspoon)

Salt (to taste)

Directions

1. Set oven to 350 F.
2. Spread pecan on a baking sheet and roast for 10-15 minutes until fragrant.
3. Put chia seeds in a grinder and grind finely; grind erythritol and combine with chia seeds in a bowl.
4. Process 2/3 of pecans to form butter, reserve the remaining pecans until needed.
5. Add eggs, nut butter, salt and stevia to chia mixture; mix together until thoroughly combined.
6. Add caramel, heavy cream, melted and baking powder to mixture and mix together then add leftover pecans and fold.
7. Grease a baking pan (square) and add batter.
8. Bake for 20 minutes, remove from oven and cool.
9. Slice and serve.

Nutritional Facts

Calories 174

Net Carbs 1.1g

Fats 17.1g

Protein 3.9g

Fiber 3.8g

Neapolitan Bombs

Makes 24

Ingredients

Butter (1/2 cup)

Sour cream (1/2 cup)

Cocoa powder (2 tablespoons)

Liquid Stevia (25 drops)

Strawberries (2)

Coconut oil (1/2 cup)

Cream cheese (1/2 cup)

Erythritol (2 tablespoons)

Vanilla (1 teaspoon)

Directions

1. Place all ingredients into a blender except strawberries, vanilla and cocoa powder. Pulse until mixture is thoroughly combined.

2. Split mixture into three parts and add strawberries to one and mash to combine. Add vanilla to another and cocoa to the final mixture.

3. Pour cocoa mixture into mold and put into freezer for 30 minutes. Remove and repeat with two remaining mixtures.

4. Freeze for an hour or more and serve.

Nutritional Facts

Calories 102

Net Carbs 0.4g

Fats 10.9 g

Protein 0.6g

Fiber 0.2g

Creamy Orange Fat Bites

Serves 14

Ingredients

1/2 cup heavy whipping cream

1/2 cup cream cheese

1/2 cup coconut oil, melted

1 tsp pure orange extract

10 drops Liquid Stevia (or the natural sweetener of your choice)

Directions

1. In an immersion blender place all ingredients. Blend until corporate well.
2. Add in orange extract and liquid Stevia and mix together with a spoon.
3. Spread the batter mixture into a silicone tray, or in paper muffins trays.
4. Refrigerate for 2 hours. Before serving remove from silicone tray and serve. Keep refrigerated.

Nutritional Facts

Calories 127
Net Carbs 0,3g
Fats 14g
Protein 1g
Fiber 0.01g

Pecan Almond Shortbread Cookies

Makes 20

Ingredients

Pecans (2 cups)

Butter (1 cup, melted)

Vanilla (1 teaspoon)

Almonds (1 cup)

Swerve (3 tablespoons)

Directions

1. Set oven to 325 ℉.
2. Place pecans and almonds in a processor and pulse until fine like flour.
3. Add remaining ingredients to mixture in processor and mix together until dough is formed.
4. Roll dough into a log and place in fridge for 2 hours or more until dough is set firm.
5. Slice into cookies and place on a lined baking sheet.
6. Bake for 10 minutes.
7. Remove from oven, cool and serve.

Nutritional Facts

Calories 194
Net Carbs 1.2g
Fats 20g
Protein 2.4g
Fiber 1.6g

Butter Pecan Fat Bombs

Serves: 2

Ingredients

8 pecan halves

1 Tbs unsalted butter, softened

2 oz neufchâtel cheese

1 tsp orange zest, finely grated

pinch of sea salt

Directions

1. Toast the pecans at 350 degrees Fahrenheit for 5-10 minutes, check often to prevent burning.
2. Mix the butter, neufchâtel cheese, and orange zest until smooth and creamy.
3. Spread the butter mixture between the cooled pecan halves and sandwich together.
4. Sprinkle with sea salt and enjoy!

Nutritional Facts

Calories 243
Net Carbs 1.4g
Fats 26g
Protein 3g
Fiber 1.5g

Choco Almond Fat Bombs

Serves 24

Ingredients

3 Tbsp cocoa powder, unsweetened

1 cup almond butter

1 cup organic coconut oil

3-4 Tbsp sweetener to taste

Splash of almond extract (optional)

Directions

1. In a saucepan over medium heat, melt coconut oil and almond butter. Stir in cocoa powder and sweetener of zour choice. Remove from heat and add almond extract.
2. Pour almond mixture into silicone candy molds. Freeze or refridgerate until set.
3. Before using remove from molds and store in a fridge in an air tight container.

Nutritional Facts

Calories 75
Net Carbs 0.02g
Fats 9.6g
Protein 0.5g
Fiber 1.22g

Lemon Meringue Tarts

Makes 2 (Serves 4)

Ingredients

<u>For curd:</u>

Egg yolks (3)

Liquid stevia (10 drops)

Butter (1/4 cup)

Lemons (2)

Erythritol (1/4 cup, powdered)

Xanthan gum (1 pinch)

<u>For crust:</u>

Whey protein (2 tablespoons)
Egg (1/2)
Salt (1/4 teaspoon)
Almond flour (1cup)
Erythritol (2 tablespoons, powdered)
Butter (1 tablespoon, melted)

<u>For meringue:</u>

Erythritol (2 tablespoons)
Cream of tartar (1/8 teaspoon)
Egg whites (2)

Directions

1. Set oven to 350 F.

2. Prepare crust by mixing all ingredients together then use hands to knead into a ball.

3. Press crust into tartlet pans and bake for 15 minutes.

4. Start preparing curd as crust bakes by zesting lemons and squeezing juice into a bowl.

5. Combine erythritol, stevia and egg yolks in a metal bowl. Heat water in a pot and place bowl on top of pot and whisk mixture until it thickens.

6. Add zest and lemon juice then add gum and whisk to thicken mixture.

7. Add butter a little at a time and whisk to combine. Place curd into refrigerator until needed.

8. Prepare meringue by beating whites until foamy then add tartar and beat mixture. Add erythritol little at a time until stiff peaks form.

9. Fill crusts with curd then with meringue and bake for 10 minutes until golden.

10. Cool and serve.

Nutritional Facts

Calories 332
Net Carbs 6g
Fats 29g
Protein 12g
Fiber 3g

Coconut Ginger Fat Bomb

Serves 10

Ingredients

1 tsp dried (powdered) ginger

0.8 oz shredded coconut (unsweetened)

1/3 cup coconut oil, softened

1/3 cup coconut butter, softened

1 tsp granulated sweetener of choice, to taste

Directions

1. In a deep bowl, mix shredded coconut, coconut oil, coconut butter, sweetener and dried powdered gnger.
2. Pour the ginger mixture into ice block trays and refrigerate for 1 hour to solidify.

Nutritional Facts

Calories 134

Net Carbs 0.3g

Fats 14.5g

Protein 11g

Fiber 0.25g

Spiced Pumpkin Crème Brulee

Serves 2

Ingredients

Heavy cream (1 cup)

Egg yolks (2)

Pumpkin puree (2 tablespoons)

Pumpkin spice (1 teaspoon)

Erythritol (2 tablespoons+2 teaspoons)

Directions

1. Set oven to 300 F.

2. Heat cream in a pan and bring to a boil then remove from heat and add pumpkin spice. Stir and put aside for 5 minutes.

3. Whisk egg yolks then add cream a little at a time and whisk to combine.

4. Add pumpkin puree and continue to whisk mixture together.

5. Add erythritol to mixture and stir together.

6. Place an inch of water into a baking dish and put ramekins into dish. Fill ramekins with crème brulee and bake for 40 minutes. Finished products will be slightly jiggly.

7. Cool for 15 minutes then put into fridge for 4 hours or more.

8. Sprinkle with erythritol and broil for 2 minutes to caramelize the tops of crème brulee.

9. Serve.

Nutritional Facts

Calories 460

Net Carbs 5g

Fats 49g

Protein 5g

Fiber 2.5g

<u>Conclusion</u>

Thank you again for purchasing this book!

Desserts are often something to look forward to after a meal. There's nothing like sinking your teeth into delectable cakes or a spoonful of mouthwatering ice- cream. However, sweet treats are often a no-no on diets and if you had ever felt pressured to avoid them then I am sure you would have enjoyed the 40 delicious recipes shared in this book.

Often we are intimidated with the idea of desserts when referring to a diet, however as you have come to know the ketogenic diet is not just any old diet. It is a most remarkable journey that I hope you will continue to enjoy. I certainly hope these dessert recipes have encouraged you to continue the journey as I'm sure you have been reaping the benefits.

I hope this book was able to inspire you to get into the kitchen and satisfy that sweet tooth without feeling guilty. I am sure everyone will be more than satisfied with these recipes.

When you make these recipes, please share them with your friends and family, let them know about the book, and encourage them not to be intimidated by the ketogenic diet. The ketogenic diet is tailored in such a way that you won't miss eating all the stuff you used to because you are still having just about everything.

Finally, if you enjoyed this book, please take the time to share your thoughts and post a review on Amazon. It's greatly appreciated!

Thank you and bon appétit!

113